Understanding Congestive Heart Failure

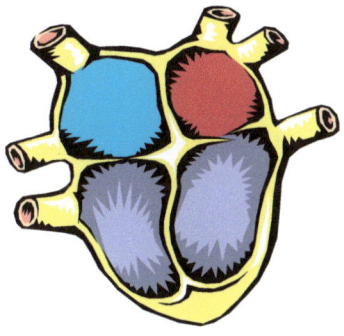

Written and Published by
Claudia Barros MSN RN CCM
7821 North 173rd Avenue
Waddell AZ 85355

For my mom, Iva

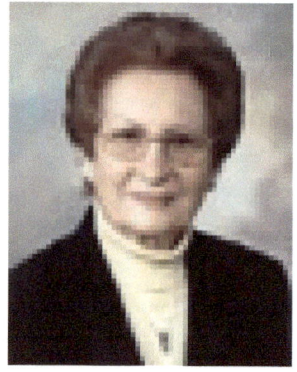

Heart Basics

Your heart is a muscle that **pumps** blood throughout your body. The **right side** of the heart pumps blood into the lungs. In the lungs, blood receives oxygen. The oxygen-rich blood travels back to the left **side** of **the heart,** where it is **pumped to your organs, limbs, and** brain. After your body uses up the oxygen in the blood, it sends the blood back to the right side of the heart and **the process** starts again.

Your heart is a complex organ made up of many parts. Each **part** plays a **unique** role in pumping blood. The heart's parts and their functions are described below:

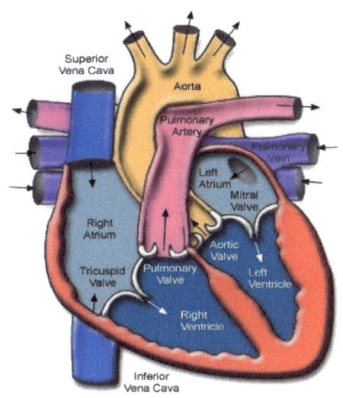

♥ **Four chambers** hold the blood as it moves through the heart. The upper chambers are called **atria** and the lower chambers are called **ventricles.** The heart muscle pumps blood from chamber to chamber.

♥ **Four valves** act like one-way doors, separating the chambers and keeping the blood moving forward. Valves open to let blood through and close to keep it from moving backward.

♥ **Coronary arteries** are blood vessels that wrap around the surface of your heart. They supply the heart muscle with blood and oxygen.

♥ **The pulmonary artery** carries oxygen-poor blood from the heart to the lungs.

♥ **The pulmonary vein** carries oxygen-rich blood from the lungs to the heart.

Fun Fact

Did you know that by the time you are 70 years old, your heart has beaten two and a half billion times?

When Your Heart Weakens

When something damages the heart, the heart muscle pumps with less force, so less blood moves through the heart. In an attempt to keep the same amount of blood moving through the body, the chambers of the heart stretch and enlarge to hold more blood. This helps keep the blood moving, but only for a while. The stretched-out heart muscle soon tires and cannot pump blood the way it should.

Because your weakened heart moves less blood with each pump, fluid backs up in the lungs. Less blood moving through your body also means less oxygen is being delivered to vital organs like your kidneys.

Your kidneys help your body get rid of extra water. If the kidneys are not working properly, excess water may settle in different parts of your body, like your lower legs. As a result, your body becomes congested with fluid, which is why this condition is called congestive heart failure (CHF).

Why Your Heart Weakens

When CHF occurs, there is usually an underlying cause. Many conditions can weaken the heart and cause CHF. Some conditions damage the heart muscle. Others make the heart work harder, weakening the heart by tiring it out.

♥ **Coronary Artery Disease ---**
When you have coronary artery disease, the blood vessels that supply blood and oxygen to the heart are narrowed. Oxygen-rich blood has a hard time moving through the narrow part of the artery. As a result, some areas of the heart muscle do not get enough oxygen. The oxygen-deprived portion of the heart muscle is too weak to pump blood like it should. Because of this, the rest of the heart muscle has to work harder to pump the blood. If too much muscle is damaged, the heart cannot pump the necessary amount of blood.

♥ **Heart Attack** --- A heart attack occurs when a coronary artery is completely blocked, stopping blood flow to part of the heart muscle. Without oxygen-rich blood, this area of the heart is permanently damaged. The damaged portion of the heart muscle loses its ability to pump, and the rest of the heart muscle has to work harder. The strained heart muscle eventually tires out and then pumps less blood to the rest of the body.

♥ **High Blood Pressure** --- Blood pressure is the force pushing blood through the blood vessels. When your blood pressure is high, your heart has to work harder. After a while, the heart's muscle walls thicken and some of the chambers may enlarge. These changes put extra strain on the heart, and the heart muscle eventually stretches and weakens.

♥ **Valve Disease** --- The valves between the chambers of your heart keep blood moving forward. If a valve does not open fully, your heart has to work harder to push blood through the smaller opening. If the valve does not close tightly, blood may leak back into the chamber, making the heart pump the same blood through the valve over and over again. Over time, this extra work can weaken the heart.

♥ **Cardiomyopathy** --- Damage to the heart muscle from causes other than artery or blood flow problems is known as cardiomyopathy. Causes of cardiomyopathy include infections (myocarditis), alcohol abuse, the toxic effects of certain drugs (such as cocaine or some anti-cancer drugs), or congenital muscle degeneration.

These diseases cause the chambers to enlarge and the heart muscle to stretch and weaken. The stretched, weakened muscle cannot pump correctly.

♥ **Other Related Conditions ---** Certain conditions can strain the heart and make it weaken more easily. **Diabetes** makes coronary artery disease and CHF more likely to occur. **Chronic kidney problems** can cause water retention, which means the heart has to pump more fluid and do more work. **Atrial fibrillation**, a rapid or irregular heartbeat, may occur along with CHF and, over time, may weaken the heart further.

Certain behaviors can also increase your risk of developing CHF. These behaviors include:

- ♥ Smoking
- ♥ Eating foods that are high in salt, fat and cholesterol
- ♥ Not getting enough physical activity
- ♥ Being overweight

CHF Facts

- ♥ CHF is a serious medical condition.
- ♥ It is one of the most common reasons people over the age of 65 are hospitalized.
- ♥ It can get worse over time and can even lead to death.
- ♥ The good news is that there are **medicines and treatments** available that are proven to help manage CHF.
- ♥ In the United States, nearly 6 million people are living with CHF.
- ♥ One out of every 5 people will develop CHF over the course of their lifetime.

How Does CHF Feel?

Common symptoms of CHF include:

- ♥ Shortness of breath, wheezing, or coughing when you exert yourself
- ♥ Weakness or tiredness
- ♥ Problems breathing when you are lying down
- ♥ Waking up at night coughing or short of breath
- ♥ The need to go to the bathroom many times during the night
- ♥ Swollen ankles or feet
- ♥ Dizzy spells

You may have several of these symptoms or only one.

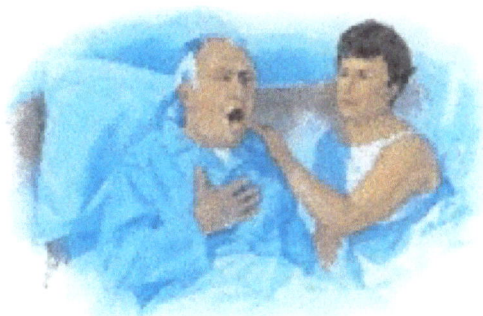

What You Can Do About CHF?

Heart failure will not go away entirely, but you and your doctor can work together to help make your life more comfortable. Your doctor can prescribe medications to make your heart work easier.

You can make some changes in the way you eat and the way you live to give your heart some extra help. Pay attention to your body and how you feel, and tell your doctor when you are feeling better and when you are feeling worse. That way, your doctor will know what kind of treatment works best for you.

Evaluating Your Heart

To evaluate your heart, your doctor examines you, asks you questions, and may do some tests. Along with looking for signs of CHF, the doctor looks for any underlying condition that may have caused your heart to weaken. The doctor uses the results of the evaluation to help develop a program for treating your heart.

- ♥ **History and Physical Exam ---** The doctor asks you how you have been feeling. Have you had trouble catching your breath? Have you been coughing? Do you have swelling in your feet or ankles? Be sure to tell your doctor if you are taking **medications for other conditions.** The doctor listens to your heartbeat and your breathing through a **stethoscope.**

♥ **X-rays,** which can show your heart's size and shape and detect any fluid in your lungs, may be taken.

♥ An **electrocardiogram** (ECG) may also be performed. The ECG will show the pattern and rhythm of your heart while identifying any irregular heartbeats.

♥ **Echocardiography** --- An echocardiogram shows the structure and movement of your heart muscle. While you rest, sound waves bounce off your heart and are converted into a picture on a screen. The test shows whether your heart is enlarged, the thickness of the heart's walls, whether there are problems with the heart's valves, and how well the heart pumps.

♥ **Cardiac Catheterization ---**
Cardiac catheterization may be
done to help diagnose problems
that could have led to CHF. The
procedure is done in the hospital
and may require an overnight stay.
A long, thin, flexible tube called a
catheter is inserted through a
blood vessel in your groin or arm
and gently guided to your heart.

Once the catheter is in place, **x-
ray contrast fluid** is injected
through the tube. Then, a special
type of x-ray, called an
angiogram, is taken. Angiograms
record pictures of clogged blood
vessels. Cardiac catheterization
can also show problems with
pumping, heart chambers, blood
flow, or valves.

♥ **Other Tests** --- Other tests can help your doctor detect problems with your heart. **Stress tests** show how your heart responds to exercise while detecting clogged blood vessels. A **Holter monitor** can help detect an abnormal heartbeat. **Nuclear scans** can show how well your heart is functioning and reveal weakened areas of the heart or blocked coronary arteries.

Your Treatment Plan

Your doctor uses the information provided by your examination and tests to develop a treatment plan. This treatment plan is designed to relieve some of your symptoms and help make you more comfortable. Your treatment plan may include:

- ♥ Medications to help your heart work better
- ♥ Changes in your diet to reduce the amount of sodium (salt) you eat
- ♥ Rest to give your heart a break
- ♥ Activity, such as walking, as recommended by your doctor
- ♥ Lifestyle changes, such as stopping smoking or losing weight

How to prevent CHF from getting worse

- ♥ Keep your blood pressure low.
- ♥ Monitor your own symptoms.
- ♥ Eat healthy.
- ♥ Maintain fluid balance.
- ♥ Limit how much salt (sodium) you eat.
- ♥ Monitor your weight and lose weight if needed.
- ♥ Exercise regularly.
- ♥ Reduce stress.
- ♥ Take frequent rest breaks.
- ♥ Take your medications as prescribed.
- ♥ Schedule regular doctor appointments.

Warning Signs

Keep alert for worsening symptoms. Call your doctor immediately if you observe any of the following:

- ♥ Sudden weight gain (2 or more pounds in 1 day or 3 to 5 pounds in 1 week).
- ♥ Increased swelling in the legs or ankles.
- ♥ Shortness of breath while at rest.
- ♥ A dry, hacking cough or wheezing.
- ♥ Dizzy or fainting spells.
- ♥ Increased fatigue or feeling unwell all the time.
- ♥ Abdominal pain or swelling.

Going to the Hospital

Sometimes, heart failure symptoms may become severe enough for you to go to the hospital for a few days. In the hospital, you will be given medications and your heart will be closely monitored.

Some of the tests described above may be performed. Based on the results of these tests and your response to the medications, your doctor may adjust your treatment program.

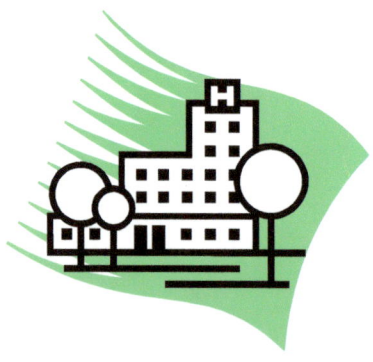

Medications for Treating CHF

As part of your treatment plan, your doctor may prescribe medications for heart failure and any underlying conditions you have. These medications may improve the way your heart pumps and relieve some of your symptoms. Some medications may cause side effects. Be sure to tell your doctor about any side effects you notice after starting your medications.
Side effects may include nausea, dry cough, dizziness, muscle cramps, or changes in your heart rhythm.

- ♥ **Vasodilators** help blood flow more easily. They do this by relaxing blood vessels and lowering blood pressure. As a result, your heart can pump more blood without doing more work. **Common types of vasodilators are ACE inhibitors, ARBs, hydralazine, and nitrates.**

♥ **Digitalis** helps your heart pump with more strength. When your heart muscle pumps stronger, it can pump more blood with each beat. This means that more oxygen-rich blood gets to the rest of the body. Digitalis can also help regulate a heartbeat that is too rapid or irregular.

♥ **Diuretics** help rid your body of excess water that may collect in your lungs or settle in your feet and ankles. Less fluid to pump also makes your heart's job easier. Because some diuretics also make your body lose the mineral called potassium, your doctor may prescribe **potassium supplements or give you a list of foods that are high in potassium. Furosemide and aldosterone antagonists are some of the diuretics your doctor may prescribe.**

♥ **Beta-blockers** help lower blood pressure and slow your heart rate. This lessens the workload of your heart. Beta-blockers may help regulate the heartbeat. They may also improve the pumping action of the heart over time.

♥ **Calcium channel blockers** reduce the electrical conduction within the heart, decrease the force of contraction (work) of the muscle cells, and dilate arteries. Dilation of the arteries reduces blood pressure and therefore the effort the heart must exert to pump blood.

♥ **Combination medications** can be used to treat congestive heart failure (CHF). **BiDil** is an example of a prescription medicine used to treat CHF that combines isosorbide dinitrate (a nitrate) and hydralazine HCl (a vasodilator). Taking combination medications can make it easier for patients to keep tract of and comply with their CHF treatment plan.

♥ **Intravenous (IV) Medications ---** Some medications must be given through an IV line. These medications work quickly to help your heart pump better and relieve your symptoms. You may also get oxygen through small tubes placed in your nose. You may have to stay in the hospital or other facility for several days while your condition is closely monitored.

Medications for Related Conditions

Your doctor may prescribe medications for other heart conditions that lead to or result from CHF. Common types of medications include antihypertensives, antiarrhythmics, and anticoagulants. These are described below:

♥ **Antihypertensives** lower blood pressure. There are many different types of antihypertensives that work in a variety of ways.

Some of the medications that treat CHF also help lower blood pressure.

💙 **Antiarrhythmics** are used to help control a rapid or irregular heartbeat. They help keep the heartbeat steady.

💙 **Anticoagulants** help prevent blood clots, which can cause a heart attack or stroke. Anticoagulants are often prescribed for people with certain valve problems, for people who have had valve surgery, and for some types of abnormal heartbeats.

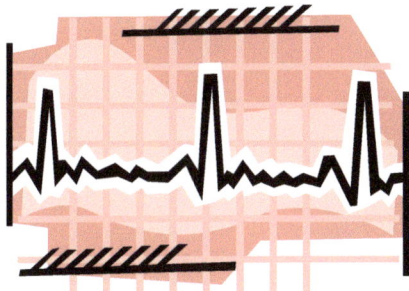

Taking Your Medication

Taking too much or too little medication can be dangerous to your heart, so follow your doctor's instructions carefully.

Even if you start to feel better, do not stop taking your medications or change your dosage unless your doctor tells you to.

Because you are probably taking several different kinds of medication, keeping track of all of them may be tricky. Here are some tips that may help you.

Have a Routine for Taking Your Medications

- ♥ Get a pillbox that is marked with the days of the week.
- ♥ Fill the pillbox at the beginning of each week, so you simply have to open each day's section and take your pills for that day.
- ♥ Take your pills at the same times each day.
- ♥ If you take them when you regularly do something else, like when you brush your teeth or eat a meal, it will help you remember.

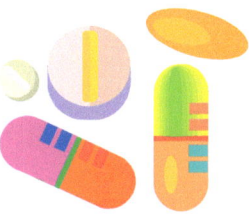

Keep Track of Your Medications

- ♥ Do not run out of medication.
- ♥ Order more medication when you still have a two-week supply of pills left.
- ♥ Carry your medications and extra prescriptions with you when you travel.
- ♥ Have a list of all the medications you take, and show the list to any doctor that you go to for treatment.
- ♥ Also show it to your pharmacist before you buy any prescription or nonprescription medications.
- ♥ Your pharmacist can tell you which medications may cause problems when taken with each other.
- ♥ Ask your doctor or pharmacist which medications should be taken with meals.

Nutrition

Eating Less Salt

Most people with heart failure need to eat less salt, which is made up mostly of sodium. Too much sodium makes your body retain water, which can make the symptoms of CHF worse. Your doctor may tell you how many milligrams (mg) of sodium are okay for you to eat each day. A common recommendation is 2,000 mg, but 1,500 mg daily is ideal.

If you have coronary artery disease or need to lose weight, your doctor may also give you other dietary guidelines to follow. Ask your doctor for a referral to a dietician to help you develop a diet plan that works best for you.

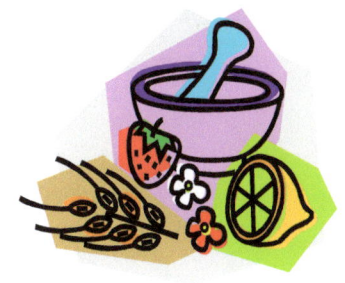

Tips for Eating Less Salt

- ♥ Take the saltshaker off the table. Replace it with salt-free herb mixes, spices, and salt substitutes.
- ♥ Do not add salt to food when you are cooking. Season your foods with flavorings such as pepper, lemon, garlic, and onion instead of salt.
- ♥ Get cookbooks containing low-salt recipes. This can give you ideas for meals that are healthy and taste great, too.
- ♥ Choose low-salt snacks such as no-salt pretzels or crackers, air-popped popcorn, or low-fat frozen yogurt.

♥ Read labels before buying canned, frozen, or other processed foods. Many of these foods are high in salt.

♥ Check the number of mg of sodium in each serving. Also, watch out for high-sodium ingredients like baking soda and sodium chloride.

♥ When you eat out, ask that your food be cooked without added salt.

♥ If you buy antacid tablets, choose a brand that is sodium-free.

Give yourself time to get used to eating less salt. You may not like this at first, but keeping your heart healthy is definitely worth it.

Over time you will begin to enjoy the actual taste of foods and not just the familiar taste of salt.

Life Style Modifications

Your heart is not as strong as it used to be, so learn to take it easy. This means getting plenty of rest and being careful not to get worn out.

There are other things that will help your heart too, like watching your weight and stopping smoking. Remember to keep all of your doctor's appointments so your doctor can monitor your treatment plan.

♥ **Get Enough Rest** --- Plan times throughout the day when you can rest and relax. While you rest, your heart muscle can also rest and get ready for your next activity. Nap, read, or just enjoy some fresh air. Put your feet up to reduce ankle swelling. Get plenty of sleep each night.

♥ **Plan Your Activities** --- Do not let heart failure stop you from being active. On days that you feel good, plan an activity like a short walk, a visit with a friend, or a little shopping. Stop and rest if you feel tired or short of breath. You will probably have good days and bad days, so know your limits and do not push yourself. Your doctor can help you develop activity guidelines or even an exercise program.

Keep moving

It may seem counterintuitive, but if you have congestive heart failure, stay as active as possible. Although strenuous exercise may overtax a heart that is having difficulty pumping, moderate exercise can actually help make your heart stronger. Other health benefits of exercise include weight loss, lower cholesterol levels, lower blood pressure, and improved circulation.

Exercises for Mr. & Ms. Potato Head

If you have always been a couch potato, it may be difficult to get moving. The good news is that even short bursts of moderate exercise can be beneficial.

- ♥ **Walk versus Ride.** Simply park farther away from the store or take the stairs down instead of the elevator.
- ♥ **Housework and gardening**. These are great ways for individuals with congestive heart failure to get some exercise as well as remain independent.
- ♥ **Walking Club.** Consider joining a family member or friend for an early morning walk around the neighborhood. To help keep you motivated, schedule a set time every day and identify goals to achieve.
- ♥ **Easy does it.** Gradually add more physical activity to your day by increasing the distance you walk or the types of activities you do.

Safe Activity Levels

Remember to avoid stressing your heart. Talk to your doctor about what activities you can safely enjoy, and what levels of exercise are appropriate for you. Ask your doctor for a referral to a cardiac rehabilitation program.

Take Care of Yourself

- ♥ **Stop smoking.** Smoking damages your blood vessels, reduces the oxygen in your blood, and makes your heart beat faster. Ask your doctor to suggest a program to help you quit.

- ♥ **Lose weight.** Extra body weight makes your heart work harder. Talk to your doctor about ways to get to a normal weight.

- ♥ **Follow your doctor's advice.** Take care of related conditions, such as kidney problems, diabetes, or an abnormal heartbeat.

♥ **Keep track of your weight.**
Weigh yourself at the same time every morning, wearing the same things. Weigh after urinating and before eating. Write down your weight each day. Rapid weight gain may be a sign that you are retaining water. Your doctor may need to change your treatment plan.

♥ **Do as much as you can for yourself.** Although family and friends may be tempted to take care of everything for you, you will feel better about yourself if you remain as independent as possible. As long as you are able, continue to be involved in managing your symptoms and making decisions about your treatment. Losing your independence can lead to depression.

Keeping comfortable

Symptoms of congestive heart failure, such as swelling and shortness of breath, can be very uncomfortable. Here are some ways you can help yourself feel better:

♥ Comfortable, nonbinding clothing and shoes may make it easier for you to tolerate the leg and ankle swelling that often accompanies congestive heart failure.

♥ Support stockings, which you can purchase at your local drugstore, may alleviate leg swelling during the day.

♥ Pillows that elevate your head at night can help you breathe easier while sleeping.

♥ Limited amounts of salt and liquids can help minimize retention of fluids, significantly lessening your symptoms.

Follow-up Visits

Start with a notebook

One of the most important aspects of managing congestive heart failure is keeping track of symptoms, medication side effects, and other concerns.

Writing down this information in a notebook will help you stay on top of any changes in your condition.

Get into the habit of recording basic information whenever possible, including your weight, diet, activity level, breathing difficulties or coughing, medications taken, and any side effects. Note any changes in your condition, including swelling, shortness of breath, or fatigue.

Finally, jot down any questions or concerns that may arise and bring them up with your doctor at your next visit.

When visiting the doctor

Most patients with CHF have many visits to different doctors. To get the most out of these appointments, bring your notebook and try to do the following:

- ♥ Prepare a list of questions before each visit. Leave spaces for the answers.

- ♥ Take notes during the appointment. If you do not understand something, never be afraid to ask for an explanation.

- ♥ If you are not following your treatment plan or lifestyle recommendations, be honest and let your doctor know. It is in your best interest to develop a realistic action plan with your doctor that works well for you.

♥ Do your best to understand all of the doctor's instructions before you leave, but do not hesitate to call the office if you have questions later.

♥ Be sure to keep all your appointments and bring a list of all your medications with you. Your doctor will monitor your condition and, if needed, adjust your medications to reduce your symptoms.

CHF PATIENT NOTEBOOK

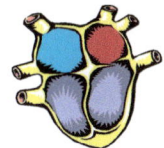

The CHF Patient Notebook can be purchased separately to help you track all of the important information related to the management of your Congestive Heart Failure.

Call Your Doctor If:

- ♥ Your symptoms get worse
- ♥ You notice new symptoms from your medication
- ♥ Breathing becomes more difficult, or you start coughing at night
- ♥ You are getting tired faster
- ♥ You begin urinating less frequently
- ♥ You gain 2 or more pounds in 1 day
- ♥ You gain 3 to 5 pounds in 1 week
- ♥ Your feet or ankles swell more than usual
- ♥ You have dizzy spells or you faint
- ♥ You have tightness or pain in your chest

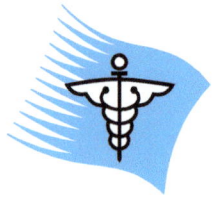

Stay on top of depression and anxiety

Depression and anxiety are common in people with congestive heart failure. Feeling unwell, being unable to do some of the things you once enjoyed, and uncertainty about the future can all contribute to feelings of sadness. If you seem consistently unhappy, you may be depressed. Look out for these signs of depression, and if you notice any, contact your doctor:

- ♥ Frequent crying episodes
- ♥ Feelings of hopelessness or worthlessness
- ♥ Poor appetite or increased appetite
- ♥ Sleeping too much or not enough
- ♥ Increased agitation and restlessness
- ♥ Loss of interest in life
- ♥ Expressing thoughts of dying or suicide

Depression is a serious problem that requires evaluation and treatment. But you may be able to help improve your moods with these activities:

♥ Stay active and connected by doing things you enjoy. Talk to your doctor about any physical restrictions you may have and discuss ideas on how to get around them.

♥ Structure your day around activities that give you pleasure and a sense of purpose. For example, plan to meet friends for lunch, or enjoy a leisurely walk through the mall.

♥ Try to stay positive and upbeat, but do not foster unrealistic expectations. Instead of thinking, "I will be hiking again in no time," you might say, "If I keep walking every day, it will start to get a lot easier."

♥ Talk about your fears and concerns. If it is difficult for you to talk about your feelings with family or friends, consider asking your doctor for a **referral to a therapist or mental health professional. A support group may also be helpful.**

Plan for the future

Having as much information as possible will make it easier for you to make difficult choices.

Depending on the severity of your congestive heart failure, you may still have many years of active living ahead. Over time your condition could ultimately worsen. As the disease progresses, talk to your family and physician about what end-of-life treatments you do and do not want. Although these conversations can be painful, it is useful to remember that these are important decisions.

♥ Find out at what point you will need or want to consider having a **do-not-resuscitate (DNR) order** added to your medical records.

♥ Talk to your family and physician about **a living will and an advanced health care directive.**

♥ You should also discuss future plans with your family and doctors. Ask about your prognosis whenever your condition or treatment plan changes.

♥ Do not hesitate to ask tough questions about what you can reasonably expect.

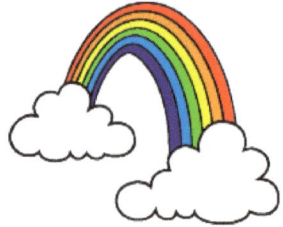

Notes: